Crystal Healing:

Guide for Beginners

By: A. R. Dupre

Crystal healing is a practice that involves using different crystals or gemstones to promote physical, emotional, and spiritual healing. It is based on the belief that these stones have different energies and properties that can interact with our own energy fields to balance and harmonize them.

Practitioners of crystal healing use various crystals and gemstones for different purposes, depending on their perceived properties. For example, amethyst is believed to have a calming and soothing energy, while rose quartz is said to promote love and compassion.

During a crystal healing session, the practitioner may place crystals on or around the body, or hold them in their hands while guiding the client through a meditation or visualization. Some practitioners also use crystal grids, which are arrangements of crystals in a specific pattern or design, to amplify their healing effects.

The goal of crystal healing is to promote balance and harmony in the body, mind, and spirit.

Proponents of this practice believe that it can help alleviate physical ailments, reduce stress and anxiety, improve mental clarity, and enhance spiritual awareness.

Crystal healing is a complementary therapy that utilizes the energy and vibrations of crystals to support overall well-being. While the effectiveness and scientific basis of crystal healing are subjects of debate, some proponents believe it offers several potential benefits. Here are some commonly mentioned pros of crystal healing:

1. **Energy balancing**: Crystals are believed to possess unique vibrational properties that can help balance the energy within the body. Practitioners suggest that placing crystals on specific areas or using them during meditation can promote energy flow, restore harmony, and alleviate blockages.
2. **Relaxation and stress reduction**: Many people find the process of working with

crystals to be soothing and relaxing. Engaging with crystals, such as holding them, meditating with them, or placing them in your environment, may help reduce stress, anxiety, and promote a sense of calm.

3. **Mindfulness and intention setting:** Crystal healing often involves focusing one's attention on the crystals and their properties. This practice can enhance mindfulness and intention setting, allowing individuals to become more aware of their thoughts, emotions, and goals.

4. **Symbolic and spiritual significance:** Crystals have been revered for their beauty and symbolic meanings for centuries. Many individuals find solace, inspiration, and a sense of connection to nature and spirituality through their use. They may serve as reminders of personal qualities or aspirations, providing a source of motivation and focus.

5. **Aesthetic appeal and environmental connection:** Crystals are often cherished for their visual appeal and natural formations. Incorporating crystals into one's surroundings, such as home decor or jewelry, can create an aesthetically pleasing environment and foster a sense of connection with the Earth's natural elements.

While crystal healing has its proponents, it also has its skeptics and critics. Here are some of the commonly cited cons or limitations associated with crystal healing:

1. **Lack of scientific evidence:** The primary criticism of crystal healing is the lack of robust scientific evidence supporting its efficacy. Most claims about the healing properties of crystals are based on anecdotal experiences and subjective observations rather than scientific studies. Without empirical evidence, it is

challenging to ascertain the specific effects and mechanisms of crystal healing.

2. **Placebo effect:** While the placebo effect can be considered a pro in terms of subjective improvements, it can also be a limitation when evaluating the actual therapeutic properties of crystals. The perceived benefits of crystal healing may, in some cases, be attributed to a placebo response rather than the inherent properties of the crystals themselves.

3. **No standardized approach:** Crystal healing lacks a standardized framework or consistent methodology. Different practitioners may recommend different crystals for the same condition or use crystals in various ways. The lack of uniformity makes it challenging to establish a reliable and replicable approach to crystal healing.

4. **Potential misinterpretation:** The interpretation of crystal energies and their effects on the body and mind can vary widely. This can lead to inconsistent

advice and confusion among practitioners and recipients. Different sources may attribute different properties to the same crystal, creating inconsistency and potential misapplication.

5. **Delaying or substituting conventional medical care:** Relying solely on crystal healing and neglecting or delaying conventional medical treatment can have adverse consequences. If you have a serious medical condition, it is crucial to seek appropriate medical attention and follow evidence-based treatments. Crystal healing should not be used as a substitute for professional medical care.

6. **Allergic reactions or physical harm:** Some individuals may experience allergic reactions or physical harm when in direct contact with certain crystals. Additionally, crystals can be fragile and may break, posing a risk of injury from sharp fragments. It is important to handle crystals with care and be aware of any potential allergic reactions.

7. **Financial costs:** Depending on the rarity and quality of the crystals used, the cost of crystal healing sessions or purchasing crystals can be significant. It is essential to consider the financial implications, especially if crystal healing is being pursued as a regular therapy.

It is important to approach crystal healing with critical thinking, an open mind, and a willingness to explore complementary practices alongside evidence-based medicine. If you have health concerns, consult with qualified healthcare professionals for appropriate diagnosis and treatment. While there is little scientific evidence to support the effectiveness of crystal healing, many people find it to be a helpful complementary therapy to traditional medicine.

Crystals have been used for healing purposes for thousands of years. They are believed to have the ability to restore balance and harmony to the body, mind, and spirit by interacting with our energy fields. If you're interested in using crystals for healing purposes, here are some tips to get you started:

1. **Choose the right crystal**: Different crystals are believed to have different healing properties. It's important to choose a crystal that resonates with you and your specific needs. Research the properties of different crystals or simply choose the ones that you're drawn to.
2. **Cleanse your crystal**: Before using your crystal, it's important to cleanse it to remove any negative energies that may be attached to it. You can do this by holding it under running water, smudging it with sage or palo santo, or placing it in the sunlight or moonlight for a few hours.
3. **Set your intention**: Once your crystal is cleansed, set your intention for how you

want to use it. For example, you may want to use it to alleviate anxiety or to improve your sleep.

4. **Use your crystal**: There are several ways to use crystals for healing purposes. You can wear them as jewelry, carry them in your pocket or purse, place them on different parts of your body during meditation or sleep, or even incorporate them into your daily routines, such as placing them near your workspace.

5. **Trust your intuition**: Ultimately, the most important thing when using crystals for healing purposes is to trust your intuition. Listen to your body and pay attention to how your crystal makes you feel. With practice, you'll learn to connect with your crystals and use them to support your overall well-being.

In the following pages, we will explore the fascinating world of crystals and their healing properties. For centuries, crystals have been valued for their beauty, as well as their ability to promote physical, emotional, and spiritual well-being. Each crystal has its unique energy and vibration, and when used in the right way, it can help to balance and restore the body's natural energy flow. From popular crystals like amethyst and rose quartz to lesser-known gems like kyanite and rhodonite, we will delve into the healing powers of these precious stones and learn how they can enhance our lives in various ways. So, let's begin our journey and discover the wonders of crystal healing together.

Abalone Shells:

Abalone shells have been used for centuries in various cultures for their spiritual and healing properties.

Abalone shells are believed to have a calming effect on emotions and can help one find emotional balance. Abalone shells are thought to have protective qualities and can ward off negative energy and evil spirits. Abalone shells are said to enhance intuition and psychic abilities, making them useful for divination and spiritual practices. Some people believe that abalone shells can help with physical healing, particularly of the heart and digestive system. Abalone shells are believed to stimulate creativity and imagination, making them useful for artists and writers.

Agate:

Agate is a type of chalcedony, which is a mineral that belongs to the quartz family. It's a popular gemstone that's often used in jewelry and has a range of healing properties.

Agate is known for its grounding and stabilizing energy. It helps to bring a sense of balance and calm to the mind, body, and spirit, making it an excellent stone for those who are feeling anxious or stressed. Agate is also thought to enhance mental function, improving focus and concentration. It can help to sharpen the intellect, making it easier to process information and communicate clearly. Agate is believed to have a positive impact on physical health as well. It's often used to treat issues with the digestive system, as well as skin problems and eye conditions. Some people also use agate to boost their immune system and improve overall vitality. Agate is a powerful stone for emotional healing. It's often used to promote feelings of inner peace and self-confidence, as well as to overcome emotional trauma and negative thought patterns. It can help to promote a sense of security and stability, which can be particularly beneficial for those who are struggling with anxiety or depression.

Amazonite:

Amazonite is a beautiful green or blue-green mineral that is believed to have a variety of healing properties.

Amazonite is said to have a soothing and calming energy that can help to relieve stress and anxiety. It is believed to help calm the mind and promote feelings of peace and tranquility. This stone is also believed to help promote communication and self-expression. It is thought to help open the throat chakra, which is associated with communication and self-expression, and to encourage honest and open communication. Amazonite is sometimes used in crystal healing to help balance the masculine and feminine energies within the body. It is believed to help balance yin and yang energy and to promote a sense of harmony and balance. This stone is also believed to have physical healing properties. It is said to help with issues related to the throat, lungs, and respiratory system, as well as with muscle spasms and cramps.

Amber:

Amber is a fossilized tree resin that has been used for centuries for its healing properties. Its warm, golden color is believed to emit a soothing and healing energy. Amber is known to be a powerful healer for the mind and body, and has been used to treat a variety of conditions.

Amber is believed to have natural pain-relieving properties. It can help alleviate pain from teething, arthritis, and other ailments. Amber is said to have a calming effect on the mind and body. It can help reduce anxiety and stress, and promote a sense of inner peace. Amber is thought to boost the immune system, helping to fight off infections and illnesses. Amber is believed to have a positive effect on the respiratory system, helping to reduce inflammation and alleviate symptoms of asthma and other respiratory conditions. Amber is said to have a rejuvenating effect on the skin, helping to reduce the appearance of fine lines and wrinkles, and promoting a healthy, youthful glow.

Amethyst:

Amethyst is a violet variety of quartz crystal, and it is a popular gemstone used in various forms of jewelry. In addition to its beauty, it is believed to have a range of healing properties.

Amethyst is believed to have a calming effect on the mind, helping to relieve stress, anxiety, and negative thoughts. Amethyst is said to stimulate the third eye and crown chakras, which can help to enhance intuition, spiritual awareness, and psychic abilities. Amethyst is often used as a sleep aid, as it is believed to help calm the mind and promote relaxation, leading to a better night's sleep. Amethyst is said to have a purifying effect on the aura, helping to remove negative energy and promote a sense of balance and harmony. Amethyst is often used as a talisman for sobriety and addiction recovery, as it is believed to help promote self-control and balance.

Angelite:

Angelite is a soft blue stone that is formed from celestite that has been compressed over millions of years. It is also known as blue anhydrite and is found primarily in Peru and Mexico.

Angelite is believed to help soothe and calm emotions, especially during times of stress and anxiety. It can also help to release negative emotions, promote forgiveness and compassion, and increase feelings of peace and serenity. Angelite is said to help with physical healing by promoting the regeneration of tissues, healing of fractures and bone breaks, and reducing inflammation. It is also believed to aid in the proper functioning of the thyroid and parathyroid glands. Angelite is thought to enhance spiritual awareness and connection to the divine realm. It can be used during meditation and energy healing practices to enhance communication with spiritual guides and higher realms of consciousness. Angelite is also believed to facilitate astral travel and lucid dreaming.

Apatite:

Apatite is a calcium phosphate mineral that comes in a variety of colors such as blue, green, yellow, pink, and purple. It is a stone of manifestation and helps with personal power, creativity, and achieving goals.

 Apatite helps to clear negativity, confusion, and frustration while increasing motivation, confidence, and clarity of thought. Apatite is said to aid in weight loss by increasing metabolic rate and suppressing appetite. It also strengthens bones and teeth, aids in the absorption of calcium, and supports the healing of bones, cartilage, and joints. Apatite is believed to enhance intuition, psychic abilities, and spiritual attunement. It helps to connect with higher levels of consciousness and can be used for astral travel and lucid dreaming.

Apophyllite:

Apophyllite is a transparent or translucent crystal that is often colorless or white, but can also be green, pink, yellow, or other colors. It is commonly found in volcanic rocks and is known for its unique crystal formations.

Apophyllite is said to be a powerful crystal for enhancing spiritual connection and communication. It can help to open up channels of communication with the spiritual realm and facilitate communication with angels, spirit guides, and other higher beings. Apophyllite is also associated with a calming and soothing energy. It can help to reduce stress, anxiety, and tension, and promote a sense of peace and tranquility. Apophyllite is believed to have a strong emotional healing energy. It can help to release negative emotions and emotional blockages, and promote feelings of joy, happiness, and contentment. Apophyllite is said to have a number of physical healing properties as well. It can be used to support the respiratory system, aid in digestion, and alleviate symptoms of allergies and asthma.

Aquamarine:

Aquamarine is a blue-green variety of the mineral beryl, and it is known for its beautiful color and healing properties.

Aquamarine is believed to have a calming and soothing effect on the emotions. It can help to reduce stress, anxiety, and fear, and promote a sense of peace and tranquility. Aquamarine is also associated with clear communication and self-expression. It can help to improve communication skills, and encourage honest and open communication. Aquamarine is said to stimulate the third eye and throat chakras, which are associated with intuition, insight, and inner wisdom. It can help to enhance intuition and psychic abilities, and promote spiritual growth and awareness. Aquamarine is believed to have a number of physical healing properties as well. It is said to be helpful for the throat, lungs, and respiratory system, and can also be used to reduce inflammation and ease pain.

Aventurine:

Aventurine is a mineral that comes in various colors, including green, blue, yellow, and red. It is most commonly associated with the heart chakra and is known for its calming and balancing properties.

Aventurine is believed to help balance and calm the emotions. It is said to help alleviate feelings of stress, anxiety, and depression, promoting feelings of peace and tranquility. Aventurine is believed to have physical healing properties as well. It is said to aid in the healing of skin conditions, such as eczema and acne, and to help boost the immune system. Aventurine is often associated with prosperity and abundance. It is said to help attract wealth and success into your life, as well as promote a sense of generosity and giving. Aventurine is believed to enhance creativity and imagination. It is said to help the wearer tap into their creative potential, promoting feelings of inspiration and innovation. Aventurine is believed to help improve communication skills, both verbal and non-verbal. It is said to help the wearer express their thoughts and feelings more clearly, and to help them connect more deeply with others.

Azurite:

Azurite is a deep blue mineral that is associated with the third eye and crown chakras.

Azurite is known to enhance intuition and spiritual insight. It is said to help the wearer connect with their higher self, promoting feelings of clarity and inner peace. Azurite is believed to help improve communication skills, both verbal and non-verbal. It is said to help the wearer express their thoughts and feelings more clearly, and to help them connect more deeply with others. Azurite is believed to have physical healing properties as well. It is said to help alleviate issues with the throat, lungs, and respiratory system. It may also help promote healthy blood flow and aid in the healing of wounds. Azurite is associated with the element of water, which is often associated with creativity and imagination. It is said to help the wearer tap into their creative potential, promoting feelings of inspiration and innovation. Azurite is believed to help alleviate feelings of sadness, anxiety, and stress. It is said to promote feelings of calm and inner peace, helping the wearer to release negative emotions and cultivate a more positive outlook on life.

Black Tourmaline:

Black tourmaline is a powerful grounding stone that is known for its ability to protect against negative energies.

Black tourmaline is believed to provide protection against negative energies such as electromagnetic radiation, psychic attacks, and negative emotions. It is said to help create a protective shield around the body, promoting feelings of safety and security. Black tourmaline is associated with the root chakra, which is the center of grounding and stability. It is said to help connect the wearer with the earth, providing a sense of stability and calm. Black tourmaline is believed to help cleanse the body of toxins and impurities. It is also said to help purify the aura and promote a sense of clarity and focus. Black tourmaline is said to help alleviate feelings of anxiety and stress. It is also believed to help promote feelings of self-confidence and self-esteem. Black tourmaline is believed to have physical healing properties as well. It is said to help alleviate issues with the immune system, circulation, and digestion. It may also help improve skin health and aid in the healing of wounds.

Black Onyx:

Black onyx is a type of chalcedony that is known for its black color.

Black onyx is believed to have protective properties that can help shield the wearer from negative energies. It is also said to help provide a sense of security and strength during challenging times. Black onyx is associated with the root chakra, which is the center of grounding and stability. It is said to help connect the wearer with the earth, providing a sense of stability and calm. Black onyx is said to help promote emotional healing by releasing negative emotions such as fear and anxiety. It is also believed to help alleviate grief and provide support during times of sorrow. Black onyx is believed to have physical healing properties as well. It is said to help alleviate issues with the bones, teeth, and blood. It may also help improve skin health and aid in the healing of wounds. Black onyx is believed to help with spiritual growth and development. It is said to help facilitate the release of old habits and patterns, and promote personal transformation.

Bloodstone:

Bloodstone, also known as heliotrope, is a dark green and red-speckled stone that is associated with the root and heart chakras.

Bloodstone is believed to have a number of physical healing properties. It is said to be helpful in treating blood disorders such as anemia, as well as aiding in the detoxification of the liver, kidneys, and spleen. It is also said to help alleviate menstrual cramps, digestive issues, and joint pain. Bloodstone is associated with the root chakra, which is the center of grounding and protection. It is said to help anchor you to the earth, and provide a sense of stability and security. It is also believed to help protect against negative energies and promote inner strength and courage. Bloodstone is said to help release anger, frustration, and other negative emotions, promoting feelings of calm and inner peace. It is also believed to help improve relationships by promoting forgiveness and understanding. Bloodstone is associated with the heart chakra, which is the center of love and compassion. It is said to help promote spiritual growth and awareness, and connect you with the divine. Bloodstone is believed to enhance creativity and intuition, making it a popular stone for artists and writers. It is also said to help improve mental clarity and focus.

Calcite:

Calcite is a mineral that comes in many different colors, each with its own unique healing properties.

Calcite is believed to be a powerful amplifier of energy, both positive and negative. It is said to help boost energy levels and increase vitality, as well as enhance creativity and intellectual abilities. Calcite is believed to be effective in promoting emotional healing and balance. It is said to help alleviate feelings of stress, anxiety, and depression, and to promote a greater sense of calm and inner peace. Calcite is also believed to be effective in promoting physical healing. It is said to help alleviate symptoms of chronic pain, arthritis, and other physical ailments, as well as promote healthy bone growth and tissue regeneration. Each color of calcite is associated with a different chakra, or energy center, in the body. By placing calcite of the corresponding color on the chakra, it is said to help balance and align the energy of that chakra. Calcite is believed to be a powerful tool for promoting spiritual growth and awareness. It is said to help the wearer connect with higher levels of consciousness and promote a deeper understanding of the self and the universe.

Carnelian:

Carnelian is a reddish-brown to orange-colored variety of chalcedony, a mineral in the quartz family.

Carnelian is believed to be a stone of creativity and inspiration. It is said to help stimulate the imagination and promote artistic expression. It is also believed to be a stone of confidence and self-esteem. It is said to help boost self-confidence, courage, and motivation, as well as promote positive self-image. Carnelian is believed to be a stone of physical energy and vitality. It is said to help increase stamina and endurance, as well as alleviate symptoms of fatigue and lethargy. Carnelian is believed to be effective in promoting emotional healing and balance. It is said to help alleviate feelings of anger, resentment, and jealousy, and promote feelings of joy, happiness, and optimism. Carnelian is associated with the sacral chakra, which is located in the lower abdomen and is associated with creativity, sexuality, and emotional balance. By placing carnelian on the sacral chakra, it is said to help balance and align this energy center.

Celestite:

Celestite is a light blue crystal that is associated with the throat and third eye chakras.

Celestite is believed to be a powerful tool for connecting with higher spiritual realms and accessing spiritual guidance. It is said to promote a sense of inner peace and tranquility, and help facilitate communication with angels and other spiritual beings. Celestite is also believed to have a calming and uplifting effect on the mind and emotions. It is said to help alleviate stress, anxiety, and depression, and promote feelings of serenity and inner peace. Celestite is associated with the throat chakra, which is the center of communication and self-expression. It is said to help promote clear and effective communication, and facilitate the expression of thoughts and feelings. Celestite is believed to have a number of physical healing properties, particularly in relation to the respiratory system. It is said to help alleviate symptoms of asthma, bronchitis, and other respiratory conditions, as well as promote healthy digestion and metabolism. Celestite is associated with both the throat and third eye chakras, and is said to help balance and align these energy centers. By placing celestite on these chakras, it is believed to help promote spiritual growth, clarity of thought, and effective communication.

Chrysocolla:

Chrysocolla is a beautiful blue-green mineral that is often used in jewelry making and has been revered for its healing properties for centuries.

Chrysocolla is believed to enhance communication and self-expression. It can help you to communicate your thoughts and feelings clearly and with confidence, making it a useful stone for public speaking, teaching, and counseling. Chrysocolla is thought to help soothe emotional wounds and promote emotional balance and stability. It can help to calm your emotions and alleviate anxiety, depression, and other emotional imbalances. Chrysocolla is also said to have physical healing properties. It is believed to help with conditions that affect the lungs, throat, and digestive system. Additionally, it is thought to alleviate symptoms associated with PMS and menopause. Chrysocolla is considered a stone of wisdom and knowledge. It can help you to tap into your intuition and access your inner wisdom and guidance. It is also believed to aid in spiritual growth and development. Chrysocolla is said to inspire creativity and artistic expression. It can help you to tap into your imagination and access your creative potential.

<u>Citrine:</u>

Citrine is a yellow to brownish-orange variety of quartz that is often used in crystal healing. Its name is derived from the French word for lemon, "citron," due to its yellow color.

Citrine is believed to be a powerful energizer and is often used to help boost energy levels and motivation. Citrine is known as the stone of manifestation and is believed to help one attract abundance, success, and positivity. Citrine is also said to enhance creativity, imagination, and self-expression. Citrine is believed to help clear mental fog and increase mental clarity, allowing one to think more clearly and make better decisions. Citrine is said to promote emotional healing and help release negative emotions such as fear, anger, and depression. Citrine is often used to balance the solar plexus chakra, which is associated with personal power, confidence, and self-esteem.

Clear Quartz:

Clear Quartz is a versatile and powerful crystal that is often referred to as the "Master Healer" due to its ability to amplify and direct energy.

Clear Quartz is known for its ability to amplify energy and intention. It can be used to enhance the energy of other crystals and can also amplify the energy of thoughts and intentions. Clear Quartz is believed to help clear the mind and enhance focus. It can help one to gain clarity about their goals and intentions, as well as to see situations more objectively. Clear Quartz is commonly used for healing purposes. It is believed to help balance and align the chakras, as well as to purify and energize the aura. Clear Quartz is also believed to have protective properties, helping to shield against negative energies and promote a sense of safety and security. Clear Quartz is often used in spiritual practices to enhance connection to higher realms and promote spiritual growth. It is believed to help increase intuition and enhance psychic abilities.

<u>Fluorite:</u>

Fluorite is a colorful crystal with a wide range of healing properties.

Fluorite is said to be a powerful tool for clearing negative energy and psychic debris from the mind, body, and environment. The crystal is believed to help improve mental clarity, concentration, and decision-making abilities, making it a popular choice for students and professionals. Fluorite is also thought to help develop spiritual awareness and psychic abilities, such as clairvoyance and telepathy. The crystal is believed to help release emotional trauma, anxiety, and depression, and promote inner peace, calmness, and tranquility. Fluorite is believed to have a positive effect on the physical body, helping to alleviate pain, reduce inflammation, and boost the immune system.

Garnet:

Garnet is a gemstone that comes in a variety of colors, including red, orange, yellow, green, purple, brown, and black. Each color is associated with different healing properties.

Garnet is said to help boost energy levels and promote vitality, making it a good stone for people who feel tired or lethargic. Garnet is believed to help ground and stabilize the emotions, providing a sense of security and safety. Garnet is thought to have a purifying effect on the body, helping to cleanse the blood, kidneys, and liver. Garnet is said to balance the chakras, promoting physical, emotional, and spiritual balance. Red garnet, in particular, is believed to help ignite passion and sensuality, making it a good stone for love and romance. Garnet is said to stimulate creativity and imagination, helping to bring new ideas and inspiration to those who work with it.

Hematite:

Hematite is a metallic mineral that is often used in healing practices. It is typically black or dark gray in color and has a smooth, polished surface.

Hematite is thought to help balance and stabilize the body's energy field. It is often used in meditation practices to help ground the body and bring a sense of calm and balance. Hematite is believed to help improve mental clarity and focus. It may also help to increase memory and improve overall cognitive function. Hematite is said to have a positive effect on the circulatory system, helping to improve blood flow and oxygenation throughout the body. It is often used to help alleviate symptoms of anemia and other blood-related conditions. Hematite is thought to help boost physical strength and endurance. It may also help to reduce feelings of fatigue and increase overall vitality. Hematite is sometimes used to help reduce pain and inflammation in the body. It may be beneficial for conditions such as arthritis, back pain, and other inflammatory conditions.

Howlite:

Howlite is a calcium borosilicate hydroxide mineral that is often used in jewelry and for decorative purposes.

Howlite is known for its calming properties and is often used to reduce stress and anxiety. It can also help to promote peaceful sleep. Howlite is believed to enhance spiritual awareness and help individuals connect with their higher selves and the divine.

Howlite is thought to promote self-awareness, helping individuals to recognize and understand their emotions and behavior patterns. Howlite is believed to be particularly helpful for emotional healing, especially in cases of anger and frustration. It can also help to improve communication and interpersonal relationships. Howlite is thought to have physical healing properties as well, including relief from pain and tension in the body, and the promotion of healthy skin, hair, and nails.

Iolite:

Iolite is a mineral that is commonly used in jewelry and is also known as the "water sapphire." It is believed to have a number of healing properties.

Iolite is said to be helpful in opening up the third eye chakra and enhancing intuition and psychic abilities. Iolite is believed to promote mental clarity and focus, making it helpful for those who struggle with concentration. Iolite is thought to be a calming stone that can help ease anxiety and stress. Iolite is believed to be a stone of spiritual growth and development, helping individuals connect with their inner wisdom and spirituality. Iolite is thought to have a positive effect on the immune system, helping to strengthen it and promote overall health and wellness.

<u>Jade:</u>

Jade is a beautiful green gemstone that has been used for centuries for its healing properties. It is believed to have a soothing and calming effect on the mind and body and is often used in meditation and spiritual practices.

Jade is said to help balance emotions and promote feelings of calmness and tranquility. It is believed that jade can help support the body's natural healing process, especially in cases of arthritis, joint pain, and other conditions. Jade is often used in spiritual practices as it is believed to help open the heart chakra and enhance spiritual awareness. Jade is said to offer protection from negative energies and promote a sense of safety and security. In some cultures, jade is believed to attract wealth and prosperity into one's life.

Jasper:

Jasper is a type of chalcedony, a mineral in the quartz family. It comes in a variety of colors, including red, yellow, green, and brown. It has been used for thousands of years for both decorative and healing purposes. Grounding and stability: Jasper is believed to provide a grounding and stabilizing energy, helping to bring a sense of calm and balance to the wearer.

Jasper is thought to offer protection against negative energies and entities. Jasper is believed to have a nurturing energy that can help to comfort and support during times of stress or anxiety. Jasper is said to have physical healing properties, particularly for the digestive system, kidneys, and liver. It may also be beneficial for the circulatory system, skin, and respiratory system. Jasper is believed to promote emotional healing and help with issues such as anger, jealousy, and insecurity.

Kunzite:

Kunzite is a beautiful pink to lilac-colored gemstone that is a variety of spodumene.

Kunzite is a calming stone that helps to soothe frayed nerves and reduce stress and anxiety. It is also believed to help with emotional healing by aiding in the release of negative emotions and promoting feelings of inner peace and tranquility. Kunzite is known to enhance spiritual awareness and promote spiritual growth. It is believed to help open the heart chakra, which can aid in the development of compassion, empathy, and love. Kunzite is said to be helpful in treating various physical ailments, such as migraines, stress-related disorders, and immune system disorders. Kunzite is believed to enhance creativity and promote a sense of inspiration and motivation. It is said to help artists, writers, and musicians tap into their creative potential and produce work that is innovative and original. Kunzite is said to be a stone of love and romance, and is believed to help enhance personal relationships by promoting open communication, honesty, and understanding. It is also said to be helpful in resolving conflicts and promoting harmony and cooperation in relationships.

Kyanite:

Kyanite is a blue or greenish-blue mineral that is often used in jewelry and for spiritual and healing purposes.

Kyanite is known for its ability to balance and align all of the chakras, especially the throat chakra. This can help to improve communication, self-expression, and spiritual connection. Kyanite has the ability to clear negative energy and blockages from the body and aura. This can help to promote a sense of calm, peace, and clarity. Kyanite is believed to enhance psychic abilities, including intuition, telepathy, and clairvoyance. It can also help to develop spiritual gifts and increase spiritual awareness. Kyanite is thought to be helpful in releasing emotional blockages and promoting emotional healing. It can help to reduce stress, anxiety, and fear, and increase feelings of love, compassion, and forgiveness. Kyanite is also believed to have physical healing properties, particularly for the throat, lungs, and nervous system. It can help to alleviate pain, inflammation, and neurological issues, and promote overall physical well-being.

Labradorite:

Labradorite is a feldspar mineral that is known for its iridescent play of colors, which can range from blue and green to gold and purple. It is often used in jewelry and is believed to have a number of healing properties.

Labradorite is said to provide protection from negative energies and psychic attacks. It is believed to create a shield around the aura, which helps to prevent energy from leaking out or being drained by others. Labradorite is often used in meditation and spiritual practices to help facilitate transformation and change. It is believed to help with self-discovery and self-awareness, and to assist with personal growth and spiritual evolution. Labradorite is said to stimulate intuition and psychic abilities. It is believed to enhance spiritual perception and to help connect the user with higher consciousness. Labradorite is often used to calm the mind and reduce stress and anxiety. It is believed to help balance emotions and to promote a sense of peace and tranquility. Labradorite is also said to be a stone of creativity, helping to stimulate imagination and inspiration. It is believed to assist with creative endeavors and to promote artistic expression.

Lapis Lazuli:

Lapis lazuli is a beautiful deep blue gemstone that has been highly valued for its healing properties for thousands of years.

Lapis lazuli is said to enhance spiritual awareness and connection to the divine. It is believed to help one connect with their inner truth and wisdom. Lapis lazuli is also associated with the throat chakra and is said to aid in clear and effective communication. It can help one express themselves more authentically and speak their truth. Lapis lazuli is said to enhance mental clarity, focus, and concentration. It is believed to help alleviate anxiety and mental stress. Lapis lazuli is also associated with promoting inner peace, calm, and serenity. It can help one let go of negative emotions and find a sense of balance and harmony. Lapis lazuli is believed to have physical healing properties as well, particularly in the areas of the throat, lungs, and respiratory system. It is also said to aid in reducing inflammation, lower blood pressure, and alleviate pain.

Lepidolite:

Lepidolite is a lithium-containing mineral that is primarily found in granite pegmatites. It is known for its soothing, calming, and balancing properties, making it a popular choice for spiritual and emotional healing.

Lepidolite is believed to help reduce stress and anxiety by promoting calmness and relaxation. It is said to help release negative thoughts and feelings and promote a sense of peace and tranquility. Lepidolite is often used for emotional healing, as it is said to help balance and stabilize moods and emotions. It is believed to help release emotional blockages and promote a sense of inner peace and harmony. Lepidolite is said to help improve sleep by promoting relaxation and reducing stress and anxiety. It is believed to help calm the mind and promote restful sleep. Lepidolite is also believed to have physical healing properties, particularly for the nervous system and the brain. It is said to help reduce inflammation, relieve headaches, and improve brain function.

Malachite:

Malachite is a copper carbonate mineral with a vibrant green color and distinctive banding patterns. In addition to its use as a decorative stone, malachite has been prized for its potential healing properties for thousands of years.

Malachite is often used to promote emotional healing and balance. It is believed to help release negative emotions such as guilt, shame, and anger, and promote feelings of inner peace and self-love. Malachite is thought to have a detoxifying effect on the body and can be used to help alleviate symptoms associated with physical ailments such as arthritis, asthma, and high blood pressure. It is also believed to help boost the immune system and promote overall physical well-being. Malachite is said to be a powerful stone for spiritual growth and transformation. It is thought to help increase intuition, promote spiritual insights, and enhance one's connection to the divine. Malachite is often used as a protective stone, helping to ward off negative energies and protect against psychic attacks.

Moonstone:

Moonstone is a type of feldspar mineral that is known for its iridescent appearance, which gives it a glowing effect.

Moonstone is believed to promote emotional balance and stability, making it a useful stone for those who struggle with mood swings or emotional instability. Moonstone is said to enhance intuition and psychic abilities, helping the wearer to tune into their inner wisdom and guidance. Moonstone is often associated with feminine energy and is believed to be especially beneficial for women. It is said to help balance hormones, regulate menstrual cycles, and support fertility. Moonstone is considered to have a calming effect on the mind and body, helping to reduce stress and anxiety. Moonstone is said to stimulate creativity and enhance one's artistic abilities, making it a useful stone for artists, writers, and musicians. Moonstone is believed to support spiritual growth and development, helping the wearer to connect with their higher self and access deeper levels of consciousness.

Obsidian:

Obsidian is a naturally occurring volcanic glass that has been used for centuries by various cultures for its healing properties.

Obsidian is known for its ability to protect against negative energies and psychic attacks. It is believed to absorb negative energy and transform it into positive energy, making it a powerful protective stone. Obsidian is a grounding stone that helps to connect you to the Earth's energy. It is believed to help you feel more centered and balanced, especially during times of stress or anxiety. Obsidian is thought to help release negative emotions such as anger, fear, and resentment. It is believed to promote emotional healing by helping you to confront and release these emotions in a healthy way. Obsidian is said to have a number of physical healing properties. It is believed to help relieve pain, improve circulation, and support the immune system. Some people also use obsidian for detoxification and to support digestive health.

Opal:

Opal is a delicate and beautiful gemstone that is believed to have healing properties in various cultures around the world.

Opal is said to have a calming effect on the emotions and is believed to be helpful for people who are experiencing stress, anxiety, or depression. Opal is also believed to enhance intuition, imagination, and creativity. It is said to help people connect with their inner selves and bring forth their creative energy. Opal is thought to have a range of physical healing properties. It is said to help with various conditions, including eye problems, infections, and Parkinson's disease. Opal is believed to be a powerful stone for balancing the chakras. It is said to activate the crown chakra, which is associated with spiritual connection and awareness. Opal is believed to enhance communication, especially in interpersonal relationships. It is said to help people express their feelings more clearly and effectively.

Pyrite:

Pyrite is a mineral that has been used for various healing and metaphysical purposes throughout history.

Pyrite is believed to stimulate the brain and improve mental function, including memory, concentration, and creativity. Pyrite is said to help increase physical stamina and vitality, making it a popular choice among athletes and those with demanding physical jobs. Pyrite is believed to have a grounding and stabilizing effect on emotions, helping to alleviate anxiety, fear, and other negative emotions. Pyrite is said to have a positive effect on the respiratory system, helping to ease breathing problems such as asthma and bronchitis. Pyrite is known as the "stone of abundance," and is believed to attract wealth, success, and prosperity into one's life. Pyrite is also known for its manifestation and manifestation abilities. It is said to help one focus their energy on their desires and bring them into reality.

Rhodonite:

Rhodonite is a manganese inosilicate mineral that is known for its pink to red color with black or brown veins. It is believed to have various healing properties and is often used in crystal healing and meditation practices.

Rhodonite is believed to help heal emotional wounds and balance emotions. It is often used to alleviate stress, anxiety, and other negative emotions. Rhodonite is said to promote self-love and self-esteem, as well as forgiveness of oneself and others. Rhodonite is thought to have healing properties for the physical body, particularly the respiratory system, heart, and nervous system. Rhodonite is said to help with meditation by providing a sense of calm and helping to clear the mind. Rhodonite is believed to stimulate creativity and enhance one's ability to express themselves.

Rose Quartz:

Rose quartz is a pink-colored crystal and is commonly referred to as the stone of love.

Rose quartz is associated with emotional healing, particularly with issues related to love and relationships. It is believed to help heal emotional wounds, soothe emotional pain, and promote self-love and self-esteem. Rose quartz is known to have a calming effect on the mind and emotions. It is believed to help alleviate anxiety, stress, and tension, promoting peace and tranquility. It is believed that rose quartz can help promote a healthy heart, both physically and emotionally. It is believed to improve circulation and blood pressure, and also to help heal emotional wounds related to the heart. Rose quartz is believed to help promote restful sleep by soothing the mind and emotions. Rose quartz is also believed to help promote forgiveness and compassion towards oneself and others, releasing negative emotions and promoting emotional healing.

<u>Selenite:</u>

Selenite is a form of gypsum that is colorless, transparent, and has a naturally reflective surface.

Selenite is thought to have a powerful ability to clear negative energy from the body and the environment, making it a popular choice for spiritual and energy healers. It is believed that selenite can help to clear mental fog and promote mental clarity, making it an excellent crystal for people who need to focus on complex tasks or creative projects. Selenite is said to help people connect with their higher selves and the divine, making it a useful tool for meditation and spiritual practice. Selenite is thought to have a calming effect on emotions, making it useful for people who struggle with anxiety, stress, or other emotional challenges. It is believed that selenite can help to promote physical healing by clearing blockages in the body's energy pathways and encouraging the flow of healing energy.

Smoky Quartz:

Smoky Quartz is a brown or black variety of quartz that is commonly used in crystal healing.

Smoky Quartz is known to be a grounding stone, helping to connect you with the earth and keep you centered. It is also believed to have protective qualities, shielding you from negative energy and promoting a sense of safety. Smoky Quartz is thought to help clear mental and emotional blockages, allowing for greater clarity and focus. This crystal is often used to promote relaxation and calmness, helping to reduce stress and anxiety. Smoky Quartz is said to have the ability to transmute negative energy into positive energy, making it a powerful tool for healing and transformation. Smoky Quartz is associated with the root chakra, helping to balance and align this energy center.

Sodalite:

Sodalite is a beautiful blue mineral that is often used in jewelry and for its supposed healing properties.

Sodalite is believed to help soothe and calm the mind, making it a useful tool for those who struggle with anxiety or depression. It is also said to promote emotional balance and a sense of inner peace. Sodalite is thought to stimulate the third eye chakra, which is associated with intuition, creativity, and psychic abilities. It is believed to help enhance these abilities, making it a popular choice for those who practice meditation or divination. Sodalite is said to promote clear and effective communication, both with others and with oneself. It is believed to help improve one's ability to express themselves, while also fostering a greater sense of empathy and understanding towards others. Sodalite is also believed to have physical healing properties. It is thought to be helpful for conditions such as high blood pressure, digestive issues, and insomnia. Additionally, it is said to have a cooling and soothing effect on the body, making it a popular choice for those who suffer from inflammation or other forms of physical discomfort.

Sunstone:

Sunstone is a type of feldspar mineral that is typically orange or reddish-brown in color with metallic flecks. It is known for its bright, sunny appearance and is often associated with the sun.

Sunstone is thought to promote a positive attitude and help lift the mood. It is believed to be helpful for those struggling with depression, anxiety, or seasonal affective disorder. Sunstone is said to help increase energy levels, stamina, and physical strength. It is often used by athletes and those with physically demanding jobs. Sunstone is thought to enhance creativity and inspiration, making it a popular choice for artists, writers, and other creative types. Sunstone is believed to help boost self-confidence and self-esteem, making it a useful stone for those who struggle with self-doubt or self-criticism. Sunstone is said to help increase leadership abilities and improve one's chances of success in business or other pursuits.

Tiger's Eye:

Tiger's Eye is a gemstone that is known for its chatoyancy, which is an optical phenomenon that creates a band of light reflected off its surface, giving it a silky, shimmering appearance.

Tiger's Eye is believed to have protective properties, shielding the wearer from negative energy and promoting inner strength and courage. Tiger's Eye is also said to help ground and center the wearer, helping them stay focused and calm during stressful situations. This stone is believed to promote self-confidence, courage, and personal power, helping the wearer to make clear, confident decisions and take action towards their goals. Tiger's Eye is also said to enhance intuition and insight, helping the wearer gain a deeper understanding of themselves and the world around them. Some people believe that Tiger's Eye has physical healing properties, such as improving digestion and reducing inflammation in the body.

Topaz:

Topaz is a mineral that is often used in jewelry and is known for its range of colors, including yellow, brown, blue, and pink. In terms of healing properties, topaz is believed to have several benefits.

Topaz is said to promote joy, abundance, and good health, as well as help with emotional balance and self-confidence. Topaz is believed to have a positive effect on the digestive system, liver, and gallbladder. It is also said to help with blood disorders and problems with the endocrine system. Topaz is said to help with spiritual growth and awareness, as well as help with communication with the divine. It is also said to have a calming effect on the mind and body, making it useful for meditation and relaxation.

Tourmaline:

Tourmaline is a crystal that comes in many different colors, including black, brown, green, pink, and blue. Each color is associated with different healing properties and benefits.

Tourmaline is known for its ability to ground and stabilize energy, making it useful for those who feel scattered or ungrounded. Tourmaline is also believed to have protective properties, shielding the wearer from negative energy and electromagnetic radiation from electronic devices. Tourmaline is said to help promote emotional balance and calmness, reducing feelings of anxiety, stress, and depression. Tourmaline is believed to have a range of physical healing properties, including improving circulation, reducing inflammation, and supporting the immune system. Depending on the color of the tourmaline, it can be used to balance and heal specific chakras. For example, green tourmaline is associated with the heart chakra, while black tourmaline is associated with the root chakra.

Let's delve into the diverse ways crystals can be utilized as powerful healing tools, allowing you to discover the approaches that resonate with you the most. Crystal healing offers a vast array of techniques and methods, each providing its unique benefits. You have the freedom to choose from a multitude of options, whether it's wearing crystals as jewelry, placing them in your environment, incorporating them into meditation, or exploring other methods. By exploring and embracing the various possibilities, you can customize your crystal healing experience and tap into the profound potential of these precious gemstones to enhance your well-being.

One common practice within crystal healing is placing crystals along the body, often on specific energy centers known as chakras. Here's a brief overview of this approach:

1. **Chakras:** In many healing traditions, chakras are considered energy centers within the body. It is believed that these

centers correspond to different aspects of physical, emotional, and spiritual well-being. There are seven main chakras, each associated with specific colors, qualities, and functions.

2. **Choosing crystals:** Different crystals are thought to possess unique energetic properties that resonate with specific chakras or intentions. When placing crystals along the body, practitioners typically select crystals that align with the corresponding chakra's energy or the desired outcome. For example, amethyst is often associated with the crown chakra, while rose quartz is associated with the heart chakra.

3. **Cleansing and intention setting:** Before placing crystals on the body, it is common to cleanse them to remove any energetic residue they may have absorbed. This can be done through various methods like smudging with sage, immersing in water, or using other cleansing rituals. Additionally, practitioners often set

intentions or visualize the desired outcome while working with the crystals.

4. **Placement on the body:** Once the crystals are cleansed and intentions are set, they are placed on or near the body, often corresponding to the location of the chakras. The crystals may be laid directly on the body, secured with fabric or placed nearby on a specific point. The duration of crystal placement can vary, ranging from a few minutes to an extended period of time, depending on individual preferences.

5. **Energetic interaction:** Proponents of crystal healing believe that the crystals' energetic vibrations interact with the body's energy field, influencing the flow and balance of energy. It is thought that the crystals' properties can help harmonize, cleanse, or activate the corresponding chakra, promoting a sense of balance and well-being.

Another common practice within crystal healing is crystal gridding. Crystal gridding is a practice within the realm of crystal healing that involves arranging multiple crystals in specific patterns to create a harmonious and amplified energy field. It is believed that the combined energy of the crystals, when organized in a geometric formation, can enhance the overall intention or focus of the grid. Different crystals are chosen based on their individual properties and how they complement each other. The grid is typically placed in a designated area, such as a room or an altar, and can be activated through intention-setting, visualization, or the use of a central crystal known as a "master" crystal. Crystal gridding is seen as a way to magnify and direct the energy of the crystals to support various intentions, such as healing, manifestation, protection, or spiritual growth. This practice offers a structured and intentional approach to working with crystals, allowing individuals to harness their collective energy for specific purposes.

Some healers will also suggest meditating with crystals to receive their benefits. Meditating with crystals for healing purposes is a practice that involves using crystals as tools to enhance the meditative experience and facilitate energetic balance. During the meditation, individuals typically hold, place, or focus their attention on a chosen crystal or a combination of crystals. The crystals are believed to emit specific vibrations and energies that can support the meditation process and promote healing on physical, emotional, and spiritual levels. By incorporating crystals into meditation, practitioners aim to deepen their connection to the present moment, quiet the mind, and attune to the subtle energies within and around them. The crystals can serve as anchors for concentration, helping to create a sense of calm, clarity, and focus. As individuals engage in this practice, they may experience sensations, insights, or shifts in energy that contribute to a greater sense of well-being, self-awareness, and inner harmony. It is important to note that individual experiences with crystal meditation may vary, and it is advisable to approach it with an open mind and personal intention while considering it as a complementary practice alongside professional healthcare.

Wearing crystals as jewelry or keeping them in your pocket is another popular practice within the realm of crystal healing. It involves carrying crystals on your person to maintain a constant connection with their energies throughout the day. The crystals are carefully selected based on their properties and intended purpose. When worn as jewelry, such as necklaces, bracelets, or rings, the crystals are believed to interact with the body's energy field, promoting a harmonious flow of energy and offering their specific healing qualities. Similarly, keeping crystals in your pocket allows for direct contact and continuous energetic support. This practice is often accompanied by setting intentions or affirmations to align the crystal's energy with personal goals or desired outcomes. By integrating crystals into your daily attire or carrying them with you, you can create a symbiotic relationship, benefitting from their energetic influence and experiencing their potential healing effects throughout your daily activities.

Placing crystals around a room as part of crystal healing is a practice that involves strategically positioning crystals in different areas to create a harmonious and energetically supportive environment. Each crystal is chosen based on its specific properties and intended purpose. By distributing crystals throughout the space, practitioners aim to enhance the overall energy, promote balance, and create a positive atmosphere. Crystals can be placed on windowsills, shelves, or corners of the room, or strategically positioned in specific areas to address particular needs. For example, amethyst might be placed in a bedroom for relaxation and restful sleep, while citrine could be positioned in an office or workspace for increased abundance and creativity. The crystals are believed to radiate their energies, positively influencing the space and its occupants. This practice offers a way to infuse your living or working environment with the supportive qualities of crystals, creating a more nurturing and energetically balanced space.

In conclusion, crystals have been used for their healing properties for centuries, and their popularity continues to grow in modern times. While scientific evidence may not fully support the healing powers of crystals, many people continue to find comfort, peace, and a sense of well-being through the use of these natural treasures.

Whether you believe in the healing powers of crystals or not, there is no denying the beauty and wonder of these natural formations. From amethyst to tourmaline, each crystal has its unique properties and energies, which can be harnessed to promote physical, emotional, and spiritual healing.

When working with crystals for healing purposes, it is essential to understand their properties and how to use them correctly. It is recommended to work with a knowledgeable practitioner or do thorough research before incorporating crystals into your healing practice.

As you continue on your journey with crystals, may you find joy, peace, and healing through the power of these magnificent stones.